Copyright © 2024 by S

All rights reserved.

No part of this book may be reproduced in any form or by any electronic or mechanical means, including information storage and retrieval systems, without written permission from the author, except for the use of brief quotations in a book review.

Table of Contents

Chapter 1: About Me: The Rollercoaster of life.................. 3

Chapter 2: This Is An Emergency Calling 999 8

Chapter 3: A New Day, A New Dawn, A New Life For Me.... 15

Chapter 4: Cooking Up A Storm..21

Chapter 5: Reversing My Type 2 Diabetes 25

Chapter 6: Study findings...32

Chapter 7: Conclusion 38

Chapter 1: About Me: The Rollercoaster of life

Hello there! Let me introduce myself properly—I'm 52 years old, a proud mum of three sons, and have called Waltham Forest home for the last 29 years. My kids grew up attending the local schools, and we've become well and truly embedded into the community. Waltham Forest isn't just a place we live, it's part of who we are. The faces on the high street, the familiar shopkeepers, the parks we've spent countless afternoons in—it all feels like an extension of our family.

Now, as for my career, it all started in the NHS, inspired by none other than my mum. She spent an incredible 45 years as a nurse—she was a force to be reckoned with, let me tell you. Watching her navigate the challenges of her work, while maintaining this incredible sense of compassion, made me want to follow in her footsteps. And that's exactly what I did. I found myself working in an East End hospital, with the elderly—yes, the elderly, not "geriatric." I've never liked that term; it feels too clinical, too detached from the dignity and richness of the lives these people had lived.

Working with the elderly was far more than just a job—it was an education in itself. They had the most incredible stories, stories that brought history to life. I'll never forget the vivid recollections of living through the 1940 Blitz, the fear, the resilience, and how they adapted to life under constant threat. And, of course, there were the stories about the notorious Ronnie and Reggie Kray, who seemed like mythic figures until I heard firsthand accounts of their presence in the East End. But it wasn't all heavy history; some of my favourite moments were when they'd turn the conversation to me. They were always curious about my life—where I went out dancing, whether I had any boyfriends, and, of course, my love for flashy earrings and watches that sparkled with every move. I could never sneak past their sharp eyes without a comment on my latest piece of bling!

Being the youngest nurse on the ward definitely had its perks. I remember our ward sister—she was only about six years older than me, but she had this way of commanding the room while still being down-to-earth. She saw that I was young and still figuring things out, and she gave me some leeway. There were days I'd roll in straight from a night out, and she'd take one look at me and say, "Take five minutes before you start." Meanwhile, the older nurses would grumble under their breath about how I was getting "special treatment." But Sister would just smile and say, "She's young, let her be." She always had my back, and I'll never forget that. We didn't just have a good working relationship; we became real friends. She wasn't just my superior—she was someone I could talk to, confide in, and laugh with. We worked hard, but we also made sure to enjoy ourselves along the way.

One of the most surreal parts of my time at Bethnal Green hospital was encountering patients with some very famous connections. One patient was a relative of Lionel Bart—yes, the man behind *Oliver!* When I found out, I had to keep my excitement in check, but inside I was buzzing. Then there was the relative of Ann Mitchell, who played Dolly Rawlins in *Widows*. Now, *Widows* was one of my favourite shows at the time, full of drama and intrigue—it had me hooked from the start. So, when I saw Ann Mitchell walk through the ward doors, I was starstruck! Of course, I kept it professional, but it was one of those moments where the line between my work and my personal life blurred just a little.

After seven years in the NHS, I felt it was time to challenge myself in new ways. I shifted gears and moved into other sectors, taking on roles in education, criminal justice, and children's social services. Each of these jobs brought its own rewards and challenges. They gave me a front-row seat to the realities of life that most people never see—the kind of stuff that goes on behind closed doors. I saw the struggles that many families face, the heartache, the triumphs, and the sheer complexity of human experience. These roles were deeply fulfilling, but they were also emotionally heavy. I had to learn to manage the weight of the stories I was carrying, and make sure I was looking after my own well-being amidst it all. When you're exposed to so much—pain, loss, hope, and resilience—it's easy to feel overwhelmed. But I learned the importance of balancing empathy with self-care, and how to process what I was witnessing without letting it consume me.

Looking back, it's been quite the journey. Each chapter—whether it was working in the NHS, hearing tales from wartime survivors, or supporting families through difficult times—has taught me something valuable. Life is complex, and no two days are ever the same. But through it all, I've kept my sense of humour, my love for life, and my appreciation for the stories that make us who we are.

Chapter 2: This Is An Emergency Calling 999

Alright, let's talk about my weight. In the Black community, a woman with a fuller figure is often described as "thick set." Now, I have to say, that sounds a whole lot better to me than terms like "overweight" or "obese." Those words have always felt so clinical, almost like a label slapped on you by someone who doesn't see the whole person. But "thick set" – its softer, more accepting, and acknowledges that different bodies have their own beauty.

My weight has always been something that fluctuated, especially after I turned 16. By the time I hit my heaviest, I weighed 19 and a half stone. Now, before you let your imagination run wild, let me just say—I still looked good! I carried myself well, and I didn't let my size define me. But, as I would later come to realise, those extra pounds weren't just about appearance. They came with some health issues that started creeping in. That's when I had to face the reality of making some serious lifestyle changes. I had dabbled in exercise and healthy eating before, but if I'm honest, I wasn't consistent with it. I wasn't taking it seriously. It was always "tomorrow, I'll start fresh," but tomorrow didn't come soon enough.

Then, in 2020 life took a drastic turn. I was rushed into the hospital with a diagnosis that threw me completely off balance. That diagnosis wasn't the end of it though—what followed was a slew of other health problems. Suddenly, anxiety and the fear of death became my constant companions. I started having these terrifying dreams where my sons would find me dead, and I'd wake up in a panic, my heart racing, unable to calm my mind. It felt like I was spiralling, drowning in a sea of information, tests, and medical jargon. There were heart monitors, endless scans, and more medication than I could count. But the worst part was the waiting—waiting for test results, waiting for answers. Every time the phone rang, my heart would skip a beat.

It was one of the darkest times of my life. But through all that uncertainty and fear, the staff at St. Bartholomew's and Whipps Cross Hospital were incredible. They treated me with such kindness and patience, even when I felt like I was losing my mind. And then, of course, there were my sons and my partner—they were my rock. They helped me see the light at the end of the tunnel, even when I couldn't see it myself. Slowly but surely, things started to look up. I thought I was finally on the mend, ready to move onward and upward. But life, as it often does, had another curveball waiting for me.

Out of nowhere, I started experiencing this unbearable vaginal itchiness. Yes, you heard that right—vaginal itchiness. I'm not going to sugarcoat it. It felt like someone had poured a bucket of itching powder right down there, and I was absolutely miserable. I was going to the toilet constantly, especially at night, scratching until my skin was raw. I felt dirty, ashamed, and completely isolated. The more I scratched, the worse it got—open grazes turned every bathroom trip into an ordeal, a painful reminder of what I was going through. I reached a point where I didn't want to see anyone, didn't want to leave my bed. I felt embarrassed and trapped in my own body. It was, without a doubt, the lowest I've ever felt in my life.

Eventually, I knew I couldn't ignore it anymore. I had to call the doctor. So, I mustered up all the courage I had and put in a request online, specifically asking for a female doctor to call me back. When she did, I explained everything—when it started, how bad it was, how it was affecting me physically and emotionally. She was incredibly kind and sympathetic, which made all the difference. She recommended a cream that she'd prescribe for me and said if that didn't work, she'd consider referring me to a gynaecologist. I wasn't thrilled about that part— just the thought of lying spread-eagle with a doctor peering down there with a bright light gave me chills. But for the moment, I was happy to try the cream and avoid that scenario.

Unfortunately, the cream only helped a little. The itchiness persisted, and I still found myself making countless trips to the bathroom at night. It was exhausting. Then, one night around 10 pm, I tried to lie down and rest, but suddenly, my head started spinning. And I mean *spinning*. I'd heard people use that phrase before, and I always thought, "How can your head actually spin?" Well, now I know—they weren't exaggerating. It was terrifying. I felt sick to my stomach, and panic set in. Something was seriously wrong, so I called my sons and told them what was happening. They were just as scared as I was.

I called an ambulance, and before I knew it, two paramedics arrived. One was so young, he looked like he could've been my son! Not that I was complaining—it was reassuring to see fresh, energetic faces. The older paramedic sat me down and started asking all these questions about my medical history. Meanwhile, I'm sitting there, head still spinning, barely able to focus. Then, the younger one told me he was going to do a finger-prick test to check my blood sugar. I was confused at first—what did my blood sugar have to do with this? But he explained it calmly and asked if I had diabetes. I told him, confidently, "No, I'm not diabetic." Then he looked at me and said, "Your blood sugar is 105." I asked him, "Is that good?" He shook his head. "No, it's very high."

That's when it hit me. Between my medical history and the elevated sugar levels, they told me I needed to go to the hospital. I wasn't thrilled about the idea, but it didn't take long for me to realise I had no choice.

When we got to the hospital, the usual checks followed—heart monitors, blood tests, the works. After a few hours, a doctor came and sat beside my bed. He was kind, but firm as he told me that I had Type 2 diabetes. The words hung in the air, heavy but not unexpected. He explained that I'd need to make some serious changes to my diet and start taking medication, specifically Metformin. It felt like yet another mountain I had to climb, but at the same time, I knew this was my wake-up call. I had to take this diagnosis seriously if I wanted to get my health back on track.

After what felt like forever, the doctor cleared me to go home. My eldest son came to pick me up, and as we drove home, I couldn't help but feel a strange mix of emotions—relief, fear, and determination. I knew I had a long road ahead of me, but I was ready to face it. And I can't forget to give a big shout-out to the NHS staff at Whipps Cross and St. Bartholomew's hospitals. Their care, with the exception of one individual who shall remain nameless, was truly exceptional.

So, that's me—a woman who's been through the highs, the lows, and everything in between. Life is unpredictable, full of twists and turns, but I'm doing my best to keep up with it all, one day at a time.

Chapter 3: A New Day, A New Dawn, A New Life For Me

Things had to change—I needed to make the changes. I knew this wasn't something I could ignore or brush off. My wake-up call had come, and I had to listen. You see, the word "diabetes" wasn't new to me. The first time I ever heard about it, I was about 12 years old. My parents had a close family friend named Sam, a man in his forties who still lived with his elderly mother. His mother was up there in age, maybe in her late 70s, and she had diabetes. At the time, I didn't fully understand what that meant, but what I did know was that it wasn't good. In my young mind, diabetes was tied to the memory of Sam's mum—she went blind, and eventually, they had to amputate both of her legs below the knee because of the complications with diabetes.

That was a powerful image that stuck with me throughout my life. At just 12 years old, I already associated diabetes with something deadly, something that could strip you of your independence and your dignity. It was terrifying. I remember thinking, "That is an illness I *never* want to have." But as life often does, it brings you back full circle to things you tried to avoid.

Years later, Sam himself fell victim to the same disease. He ended up in the same tragic situation as his mother—blind and with amputations—before succumbing to complications of diabetes. It shook me to the core. It was like a cruel cycle that ran in their family, and I feared the same could happen to me if I wasn't careful.

So, when I got my diagnosis, all those childhood memories came flooding back. For the first few days after finding out I had Type 2 diabetes, I was scared, lost, and completely unsure about what to do. Everything I wanted to eat or drink, I'd find myself nervously googling: "Can you eat this if you have diabetes?" or "Is it safe for diabetics to drink this?" It was as if I no longer trusted my own instincts when it came to food. Every little thing felt like a potential threat to my health.

Around the same time, the doctors contacted me to let me know that my prescription for metformin was ready, and I should start taking it immediately. Thankfully, my local chemist delivers medication, so I didn't even have to go out and pick it up. That was a relief because I was still dealing with the itchiness that had taken over my life, later realising that the itchiness was a symptom of diabetes.

I then received a letter to attend an eye screening appointment, followed by a call from my doctors asking me to make an appointment for a Diabetic check.

I started taking the metformin and thought, "Okay, this should be fine. No side effects so far." But, oh boy, I spoke too soon. The very next day, I had to rush to the toilet with severe diarrhoea and a stomach ache that wouldn't quit. I remember thinking, "This can't be happening." But, sure enough, the information on the medication said that diarrhoea was a common side effect. I tried to be patient, convincing myself that it would ease up after a few days. Maybe my body just needed to adjust.

Well, let me tell you, patience didn't help. Days turned into weeks, and the diarrhoea just wouldn't let up. It was relentless. I'd be out running errands or trying to go about my day, and suddenly, I'd have to dash to the nearest public toilet. On more than one occasion, I barely made it in time, and a few times, I almost had a serious accident in public. I can't even begin to describe the humiliation and anxiety that came with that.

It got to the point where I became too scared to leave the house. I started mapping out my every move—planning my journeys based on where the nearest toilets were, how long it would take to get from point A to point B, and when I thought the next "bout" might hit. It was exhausting, mentally and physically. I'd cancel appointments, avoid social gatherings, and just stay home because I couldn't bear the thought of being caught off-guard. I felt trapped in my own body, and my life became so restricted that I barely recognised it anymore. I was living like a hermit, afraid to step out of my front door.

After months of this, I couldn't take it anymore. I called my doctor and told him point-blank, "I can't keep doing this. This medication is ruining my life." He suggested switching me to a slow-release version of metformin, hoping that would help with the side effects. But unfortunately, that didn't work either. The diarrhoea continued, and so did my misery. I knew I couldn't keep living like this. Something had to give.

Finally, I spoke to my doctor again, and this time, she really listened to me. She could hear the frustration and desperation in my voice. I explained how the metformin was making it impossible for me to live a normal life, how I was too afraid to go anywhere because of the constant fear of an "accident." Thankfully, she understood my plight and agreed that it wasn't working for me. She allowed me to stop taking the metformin and assured me that we'd find another way to manage my diabetes.

Once I stopped the metformin, things began to improve. I still had my other medications, and with those, I was able to keep my diabetes under control without the awful side effects. It felt like a huge weight had been lifted off my shoulders. I was finally able to step out of the house without that constant fear lurking in the back of my mind. Little by little, I started reclaiming my life, getting back to a routine that felt more like me.

This journey has been far from easy, and there are still days when I struggle, but I've learned that managing diabetes isn't just about the medication—it's about understanding your body, your limits, and finding what works for you. Sometimes that means standing up for yourself, pushing back when something isn't right, and being your own advocate.

It's not just about surviving with diabetes—it's about living well with it. And I'm determined to do just that.

Chapter 4: Cooking Up A Storm

This chapter is all about the culinary adventures I embarked on while revamping my diet. Let me tell you, it was quite the tasty journey! Now, I'll admit, sweet potatoes and I didn't get off to a great start. They weren't my favourite at first, but after some creative experimentation, I stumbled upon a recipe that made me a believer. Here's my secret: grab half a small sweet potato, grate it, and squeeze out the juice (yes, really!). Do the same with a small onion and carrot—feel free to toss in any other veggies you like. Mix it all up with a bit of water and whole grain flour, lightly fry it, and voilà! The result? Pure gorgeousness on a plate.

And then there's mushrooms—my personal fave. Now, I know mushrooms can be a bit divisive, but for me, stuffing them with garlic and cheese is nothing short of a divine experience. It's like a little piece of heaven in every bite.

As part of my transformation, I also became a wholegrain devotee. There's just something about that extra fibre and texture that left me feeling full and satisfied. Now, let's talk chicken. Oh boy, do I love chicken. Through this process, I've become a pro at cooking it in all kinds of ways. My current obsession? Stuffing chicken with herbs and roasting it to perfection. And grilled chicken with a medley of seasonings? Mouthwateringly moorish, if I do say so myself.

Fish was an essential part of my diet, i began to eat salmon, mackerel, Tuna fish, which was always eaten with vegetables or salad. My favourite was salmon baked in sweet chilli sauce.

Ah, avocado! What can I say besides "love it, love it, LOVE it!" I've become quite the avocado addict, enjoying one every day—whether it's on a slice of brown bread or nestled in a seeded bun. It's my little green piece of happiness.

I am a lover of fruits so to incorporate more fruits in my diet was very easy for, I love the blueberries, blackberries and strawberries, I wasn't keen on raspberry though.

Now, I know what you're thinking: these foods might sound a bit, well, bland. But trust me, there are endless ways to spice things up. A dash of seasonings here, a sprinkle of herbs there, and adding vibrant veggies and fresh salads makes even the simplest dish look like a colourful feast.

And hey, I get it—there are foods you may not be thrilled about. But give them a shot! You never know, you might surprise yourself, just like I did with sweet potatoes and other foods I once turned my nose up at. Vegetables may not be the most popular kids at the food party, but they are absolute VIPs when it comes to a healthy diet. So, do yourself a favour and invite them into your meals—you won't regret it!

Chapter 5: Reversing My Type 2 Diabetes

When I first started taking medication for Type 2 diabetes, it was overwhelming. I had so many questions, so much uncertainty, and I felt a deep need to connect with someone—anyone—who could share in my experience. I craved a sense of community, and looking back, I wish I had known about diabetes workshops or support groups. The chance to speak with others going through the same struggles would have been invaluable at that time. Instead, I had to navigate much of the journey on my own.

For the next seven months, I made it my mission to reverse my diabetes. It wasn't an easy road by any stretch of the imagination. I had to dive deep into research, create a plan that worked for me, and find the strength to stick with it, even on the hardest days. One of the most significant changes I made was around my food choices. Coming from a Caribbean background, my diet had always been rich in foods that were heavy in carbohydrates—delicious, yes, but not the best for managing diabetes. I knew I couldn't just give up everything I loved, so I focused on moderation. I learned that I could still enjoy some of my favourite Caribbean dishes but in much smaller portions and balanced with healthier options like vegetables and salads.

Another key change was how much water I drank. You hear it all the time, "Drink more water," but I didn't realise how much of a difference it could make until I started paying attention. Hydration became a crucial part of my routine, and it helped with both my physical health and my mental clarity.

Exercise was another challenge. I've never been the kind of person to enjoy a strict workout regimen, but I knew I had to incorporate more movement into my life. I started small, with regular walks. Gradually, I built up my stamina and added in more structured exercises. At first, I doubted whether I could stick to it, but as time went on, I realised how much better I felt—both physically and mentally. This wasn't just about reversing diabetes; it was about transforming my entire approach to health.

Around the five-month mark, I felt like I was making real progress, so I contacted my doctor and requested another blood test to check my sugar levels. I had put in so much effort, and I was eager to see if my hard work was paying off. When the results came in, I was both nervous and excited. The wait felt like forever. Finally, three weeks later, I got the call: my HbA1c levels had dropped from a staggering 105 to 35. I was ecstatic! I couldn't believe it. I had done it. The doctor was just as thrilled, congratulating me on what he called a remarkable achievement. His encouragement meant the world to me, and for the first time in a long time, I felt truly proud of myself.

A few months later, I received an unexpected call from the receptionist at my GP's surgery. They were setting up a diabetes group workshop, and they wanted to know if I'd be willing to give a talk about my experience. I was taken aback but immediately agreed. This was exactly the kind of opportunity I had wished for during my own journey. A week later, I was contacted by Alex Kriados, the group leader and Health & Wellbeing Coach. She told me that my story could inspire others and that sharing my journey would make a huge difference. Her words filled me with both nerves and excitement.

The day of the workshop arrived, and I was nervous. Standing in front of a group of 12 people, all facing their own battles with diabetes, felt daunting. But once I started talking, the words just flowed. I explained how I had reversed my Type 2 diabetes and the steps I took to get there. By the end, the group applauded and congratulated me. It felt incredible to know that my story had resonated with them. Many of them asked me questions about my food choices, the exercises I did, and how I stayed motivated. That interaction led to new friendships—shoutout to Beverley and Angela!—and a sense of community I hadn't realised I'd been missing.

One person who really stood out to me was Alex. She was a source of constant support and encouragement, not just for me but for the entire group. She introduced me to techniques I hadn't considered before—like breathing exercises and self-love practices—which became crucial for my ongoing journey of maintaining my health and mindset. Her "Women's Self-Love & Vibration" sessions helped me not only manage my diabetes but also deal with the emotional baggage I had been carrying for years. She taught me how to focus on my thoughts, control my triggers, and remain positive, even when things seemed tough.

Through those sessions, I began to unpack a lot of unresolved feelings—anger, betrayal, and rejection—that had weighed me down for so long. I realised I had been holding onto things that were preventing me from fully embracing the new, stronger version of myself. With Alex's help, I was able to release that pain, and for the first time in my life, I felt free to move on from my past. I started to rediscover who I was at my core: a happy, vibrant woman, full of passion and care. The transformation wasn't just physical—it was emotional and spiritual. I was healing from the inside out.

My mum used to say, "Nothing happens before its time," and looking back, I think she was right. Although I wish I had found a support group while I was in the thick of my journey, things worked out in the end. If I had gone to a group back then, I might have found comfort in sharing my fears and frustrations with others who were going through the same thing. But perhaps I wasn't ready for that level of vulnerability at the time. In the end, meeting Alex and participating in her sessions allowed me to finally put things in perspective and manage my emotions. It taught me that healing is not just about the body—it's about the mind and the soul too. In a way, it *was* the right time after all.

Now, nearly two years later, I am proud to say that I am still diabetes-free. I feel amazing, in control, and at peace with myself. I've learned to trust in my journey, and I know that whatever comes next, I have the tools, the support, and the strength to face it head-on.

Chapter 6: Study findings

In 2022, I conducted a diabetes study that involved 50 participants, each with their own unique journey and challenges in managing diabetes. Out of the 50 participants, 49 were diagnosed with Type 2 diabetes, and only one had Type 1 diabetes. The study aimed to explore the diverse experiences of people living with diabetes, from how they managed their condition to the physical and emotional toll it had on their lives.

The ages of the participants ranged from 16 to 79 years, showcasing how diabetes affects people of all ages. Interestingly, the majority of the participants—45 of them—came from ethnic minority backgrounds, with just five identifying as Caucasian. Of the total group, 32 were women and 18 were men. Most of the participants had been living with Type 2 diabetes for over five years, and some for as long as 10 or even 20 years. In fact, only three participants had been diagnosed within the last four years.

Medication was a significant part of the study. Forty-five participants were taking metformin, a common medication for Type 2 diabetes, while five were on insulin. Unfortunately, diabetes had taken a more severe toll on some individuals. Two male participants and one female had experienced amputations due to complications from their diabetes—one had their leg amputated below the knee, and the other two had lost a toe. One female participant was on dialysis and awaiting a kidney transplant. Heartbreakingly, two participants passed away due to complications related to their diabetes.

One of the most striking findings was the lack of lifestyle changes among the participants. A vast number of them were still consuming high proportions of foods that raised their blood sugar levels, and very few were controlling their portion sizes. This was concerning, as dietary management is crucial for managing diabetes.

When it came to exercise, only a small handful of participants reported doing any form of physical activity, such as going for walks. Exercise, even something as simple as walking, can significantly help manage blood sugar levels and improve overall health, but many participants were not incorporating it into their routines.

What was even more alarming was the participants' inconsistent use of their medication. Roughly half of the group was taking their prescribed dosage as recommended by their doctors, while the other half admitted to taking their medication sporadically, if at all. Many participants shared that they weren't taking their medication regularly due to the unpleasant side effects they experienced, such as diarrhoea, headaches, vision problems, and issues with their feet. These side effects, unfortunately, led some to stop their medication altogether, which only worsened their symptoms and long-term health prospects.

Through this study, I was able to learn so much more about how individuals manage—or, in many cases, struggle to manage—their diabetes. While I had reversed my own Type 2 diabetes within seven months, hearing the experiences of others gave me a deeper understanding of how complicated and challenging diabetes can be, especially for those who may not have access to the same resources or support that I did.

One of the most surprising findings from my study was that nearly half of the participants didn't take immediate action when they were first told they were pre-diabetic or diagnosed with Type 2 diabetes. Some of them waited months or even years before making any significant lifestyle changes. This delay in action was shocking to me, given the serious consequences of unmanaged diabetes. Several participants said they had been in denial about their diagnosis, thinking they could continue with their usual routines without significant repercussions. Unfortunately, by the time some of them began to take their condition seriously, they were already dealing with severe complications, including amputations, kidney failure, and vision loss.

One of the most important lessons I took away from this study is how vital it is to make lifestyle changes as soon as you receive a diabetes diagnosis—or even when you are told you're at risk. Diabetes is a serious condition that can lead to devastating health problems if not managed properly. The study highlighted the tragic outcomes of not taking your medication as prescribed and failing to make necessary changes, such as adjusting your diet and incorporating exercise into your life.

If you're diagnosed with diabetes or are pre-diabetic, it's critical to understand that this is not a condition you can afford to ignore. Even if the medication you've been prescribed causes unpleasant side effects, it's essential to communicate with your doctor. Many participants in my study weren't aware that there are often alternative medications available or that their dosage could be adjusted to reduce side effects. Instead of suffering in silence or stopping your medication altogether, it's crucial to speak up. Your doctor can help find a solution that works for you, whether it's a different medication or a lower dosage that reduces the impact of side effects.

The stories of those I spoke with during this study have left a lasting impression on me. While I was able to reverse my own diabetes, I know that managing this condition is a long-term journey, one that requires consistent effort and determination. I am grateful to the 50 participants who shared their personal stories and struggles with me. Through them, I've learned that no two diabetes journeys are the same, but the need for awareness, education, and support is universal. Whether you're newly diagnosed or have been living with diabetes for years, taking control of your health is always within your reach—it's never too late to make a change.

Chapter 7: Conclusion

I want to take a moment to express my deepest gratitude to everyone who has stood by me through the ups and downs of my journey with my medical conditions, particularly in reversing my Type 2 diabetes. This journey has been long and, at times, incredibly challenging, but I wouldn't have made it through without the love, support, and strength of those around me.

A massive shout-out goes to my three incredible sons, N'yahh, Jah'heim, and Zy'On. You have been my unwavering pillars of strength, my rock, through it all. You're constant support, your words of encouragement, and even just the quiet moments where you stood by me in my most difficult times, have been the greatest source of healing for me. There were days when I didn't think I could push through, when the fear and uncertainty of my health weighed heavily on me, but you never let me give up. You reminded me of the fighter I am, and for that, I will forever be grateful.

Watching you grow into the strong, caring, and resilient individuals that you are has been my greatest joy, and I am so proud to call you my sons. You not only gave me the courage to fight for my health but also the motivation to strive for better, to never settle for less than I deserve. I know I couldn't have reversed my diabetes without the three of you by my side, holding me up when I felt weak and celebrating with me when I hit milestones. Your love has been my greatest gift, and I hope you know how much it means to me.

To everyone else who has been part of my journey—my family, friends, doctors, nurses, and all the amazing people who have helped along the way—thank you from the bottom of my heart. It's because of your guidance, patience, and care that I was able to make the changes necessary to take control of my health. Whether you offered advice, lent a listening ear, or simply believed in me when I didn't believe in myself, your support made all the difference.

As I reflect on my own journey, I want to extend my heartfelt wishes to all of you who are on your own path, whether you are working to reverse your diabetes or striving to manage it successfully. I understand the fears, the frustrations, and the uncertainties that come with living with diabetes, but I also know that with the right mindset, determination and support, you can achieve incredible things. It may not be easy, and there will be challenges, but remember that every step forward is a victory in of itself. You are stronger than you know, and I truly believe that each of you can overcome this, just as I have.

To those who are just beginning their journey with diabetes, I wish you strength and perseverance. It's a process, and it can feel overwhelming at times, but don't lose hope. Educate yourself, lean on those around you, and never be afraid to ask for help. You are not alone in this fight, and there is always a way forward, even when the road feels rough.

For those who are managing diabetes day by day, I wish you continued success in maintaining your health. Your resilience is admirable, and I hope you take pride in every small victory you achieve, whether it's improving your diet, sticking to your exercise routine, or managing your blood sugar levels. Every effort you make is a testament to your strength and commitment to living a healthier, happier life.

My journey with diabetes has taught me that healing is not just about the physical body; it's about the mind, heart, and soul as well. Surround yourself with love, with positivity, and with people who believe in your ability to succeed. Trust in your own strength, and never underestimate the power of hope and perseverance.

I send you all my love, success, and best wishes as you continue on your journey. Whether you are aiming to reverse your diabetes or simply manage it more effectively, know that you have the power within you to make it happen. Stay focused, stay determined, and most importantly, stay hopeful. You've got this.